Godya™

God's Yoga for Kids

I0135471

Godya

God's Yoga for Kids

Copyright © 2021 by Digital Designz, Inc.

By Linda Sakevich, illustrated by Nikki Boetger and designed by Charles John Sakevich

All rights reserved. No portion of this book may be reproduced, stored in a retrieval system, or transmitted in any form or by any means - electronic, mechanical, photocopy, recording, scanning or other - except for brief quotations in critical reviews or articles, without the prior written permission of the publisher.

Scripture quotations marked (ESV) are from The ESV® Bible (The Holy Bible, English Standard Version®), copyright © 2001 by Crossway, a publishing ministry of Good News Publishers. Used by permission. All rights reserved.

The Holy Bible: International Standard Version. Release 2.0, Build 2015.02.09. Copyright © 1995-2014 by ISV Foundation. All rights reserved internationally. Used by permission of Davidson Press, LLC.

Scriptures taken from the Holy Bible, New International Version®, NIV®. Copyright © 1973, 1978, 1984, 2011 by Biblica, Inc.™. Used by permission of Zondervan. All rights reserved worldwide. www.zondervan.com The "NIV" and "New International Version" are trademarks registered in the United States Patent and Trademark Office by Biblica, Inc.™

Digital DesignZ Inc.

Published by Digital Designz, Inc.

Godya is a registered trademark of Digital Designz, Inc.

Godya™ Titles may be purchased in bulk for educational, business, fund-raising, or sales promotional use.

For more information, please email info@Godya.net.

ISBN 978-1-7367600-2-4

ISBN 978-1-7367600-1-7 (electronic)

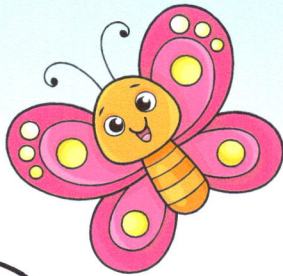

Godya™
God's Yoga for Kids
Animal Shapes

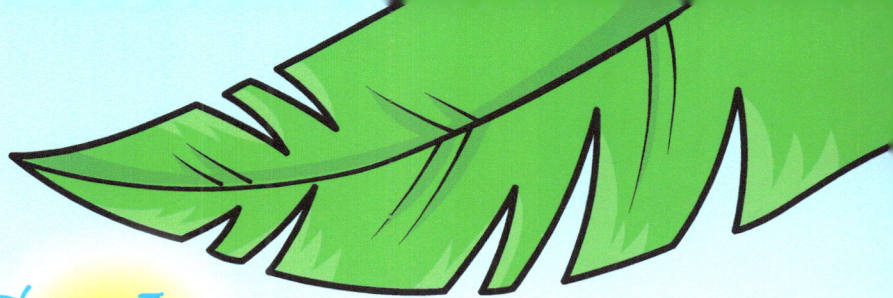

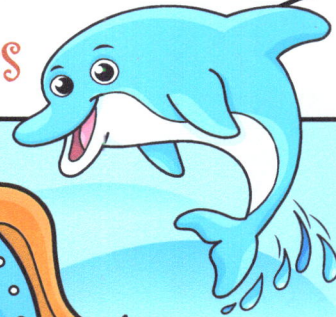

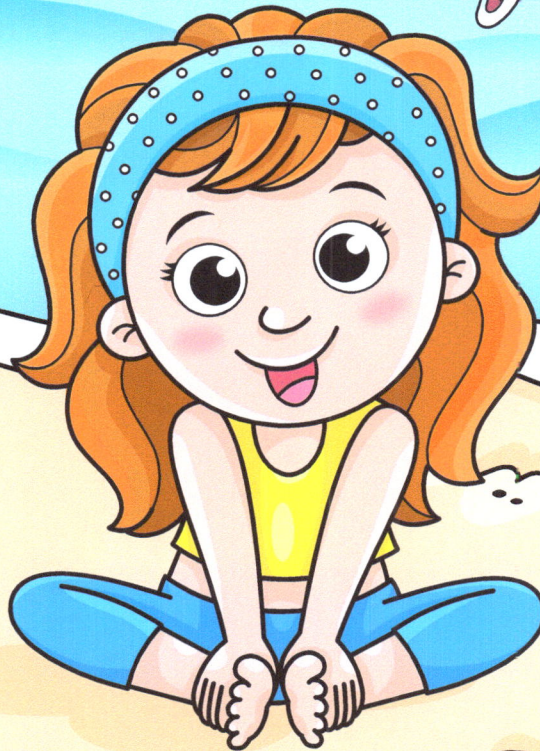

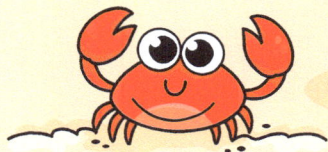

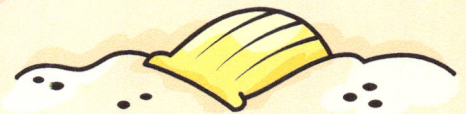

Godya is a book of yoga
animal shapes and bible verses.
Each animal has a shape, sound
and related verse. Its a fun way
to learn yoga for young children
ages two to six.

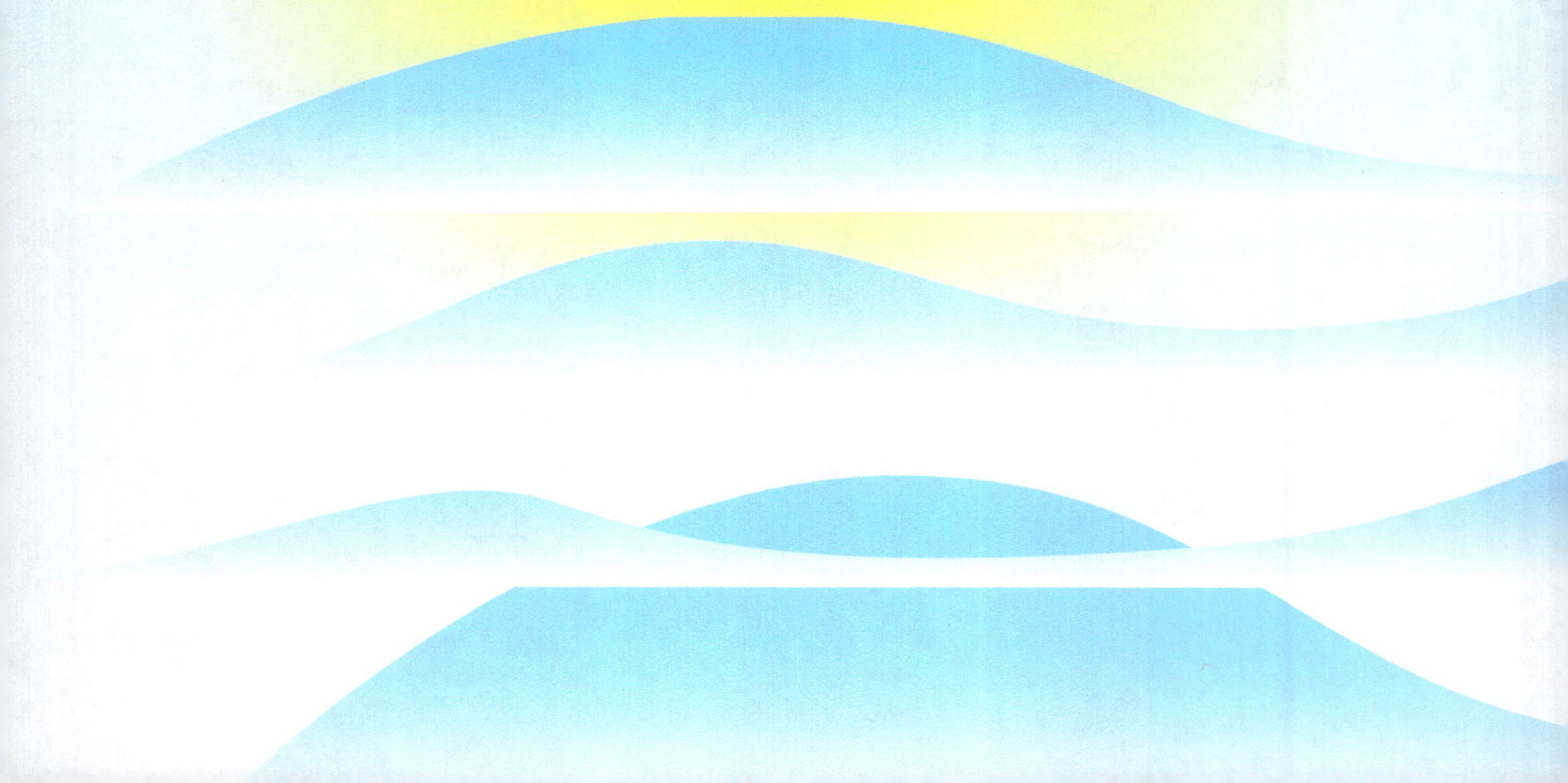

And God said,
"Let the land produce living creatures
according to their kinds: the livestock,
the creatures that move along the
ground, and the wild animals,
each according to its kind."

Genesis 1:24

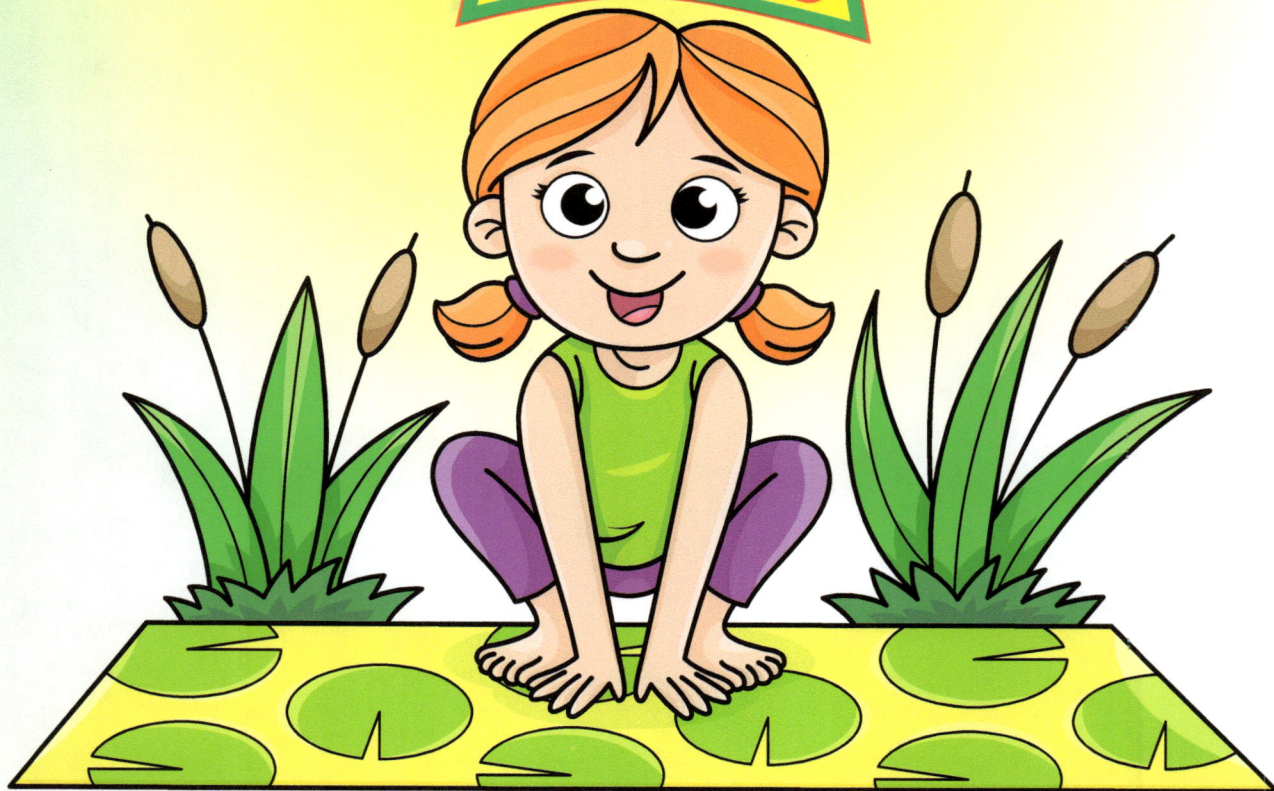

Frog
SHAPE

Place feet wide and lower hips into a squat.
Then lower your hands to the floor between your legs.

Can you "Ribbit" like a Frog?

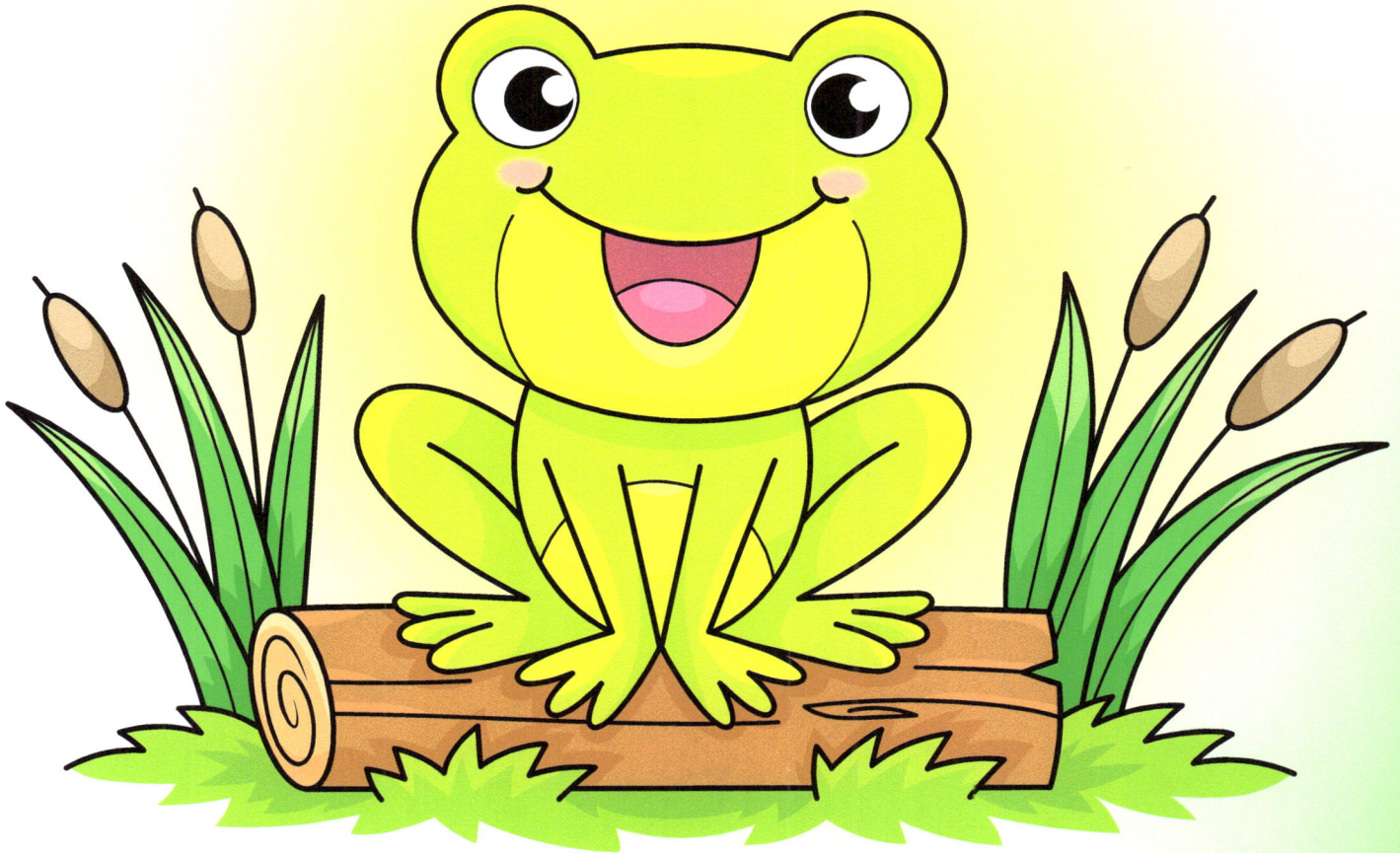

So Aaron stretched out his hand over the
waters of Egypt, and the frogs came up...
Exodus 8:6 ESV

Butterfly

SHAPE

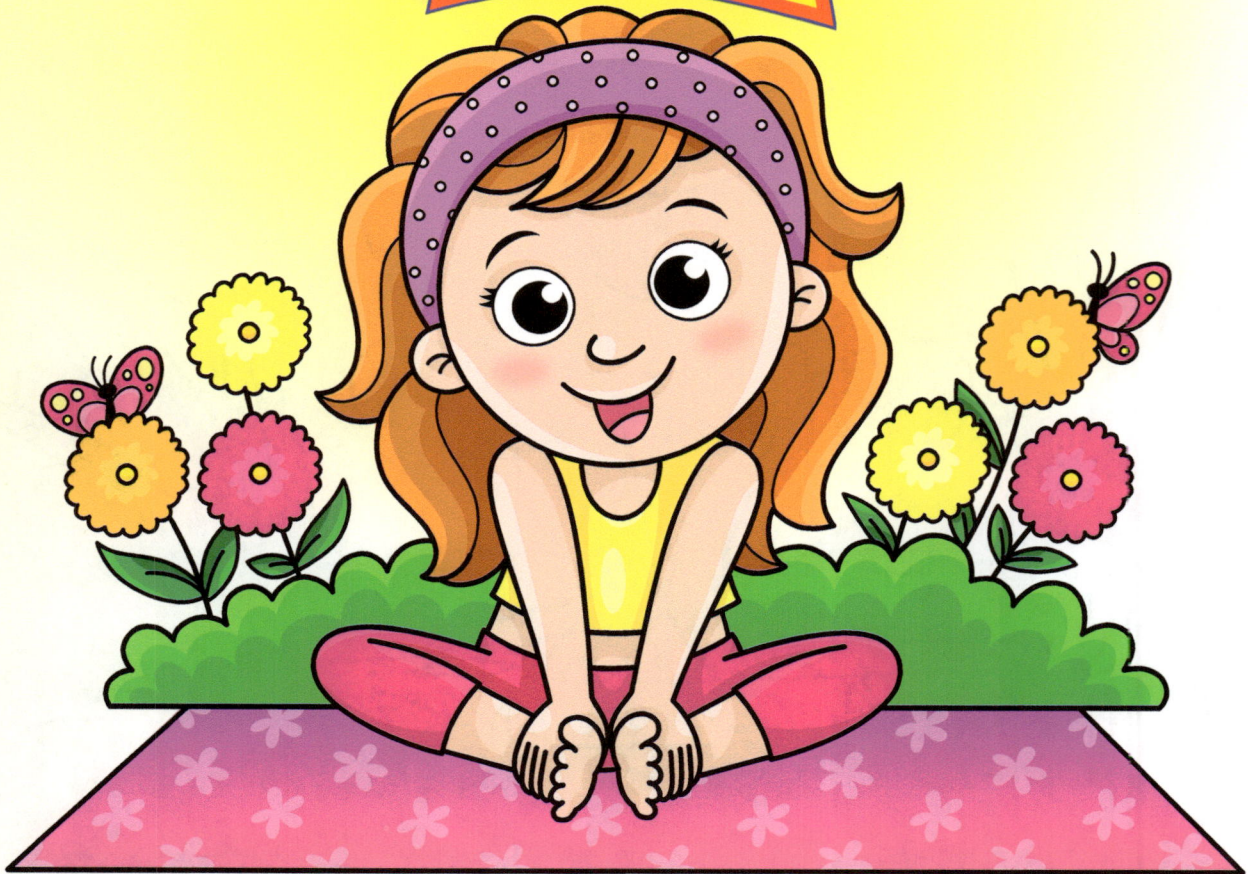

Sit up straight and bend your legs,
so that your bottom of your feet touch.

Can you "Fly" like a Butterfly?

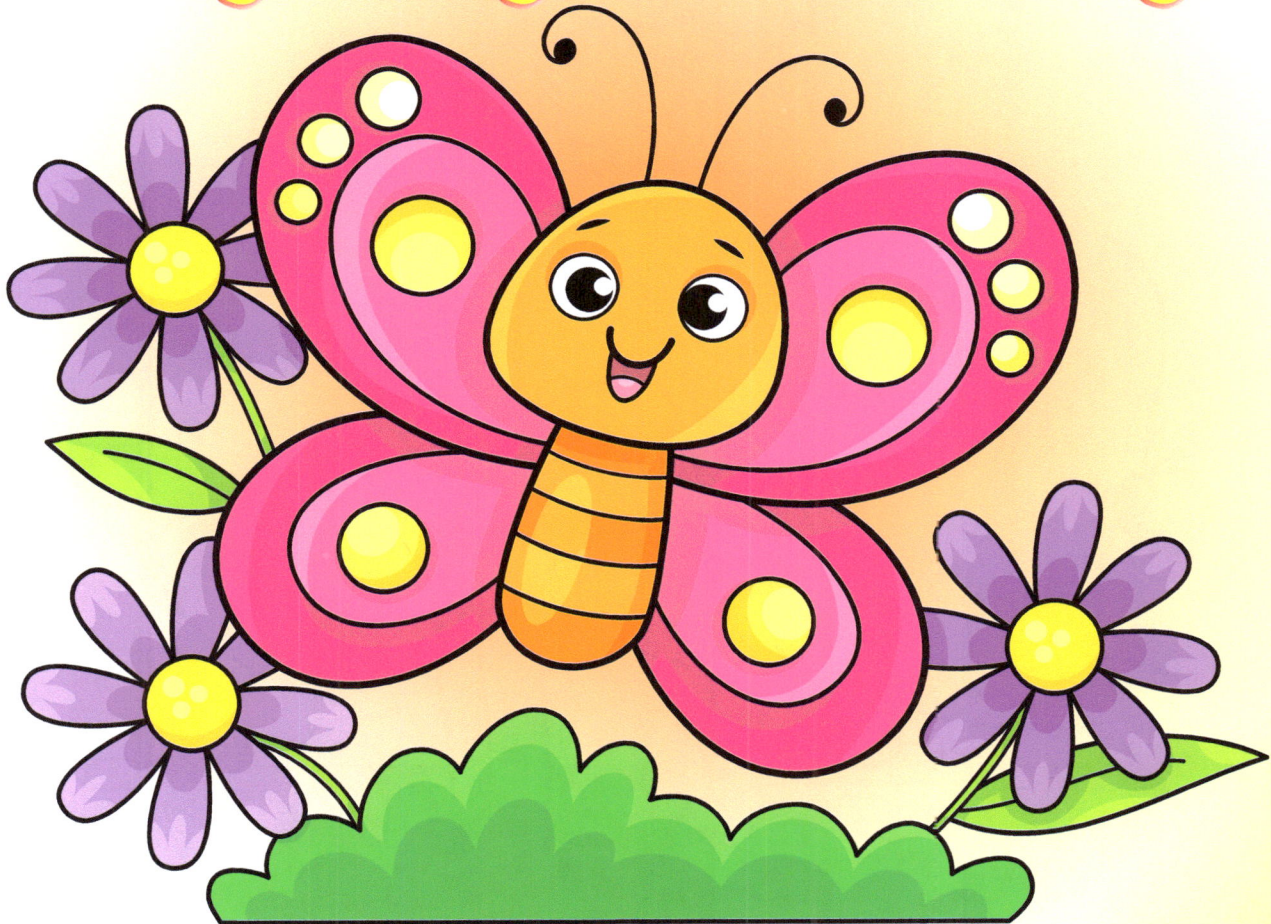

Therefore, if anyone is in Christ,
the new creation has come.

(caterpillar to butterfly)

2 Corinthians 5:17 NIV

Cat
SHAPE

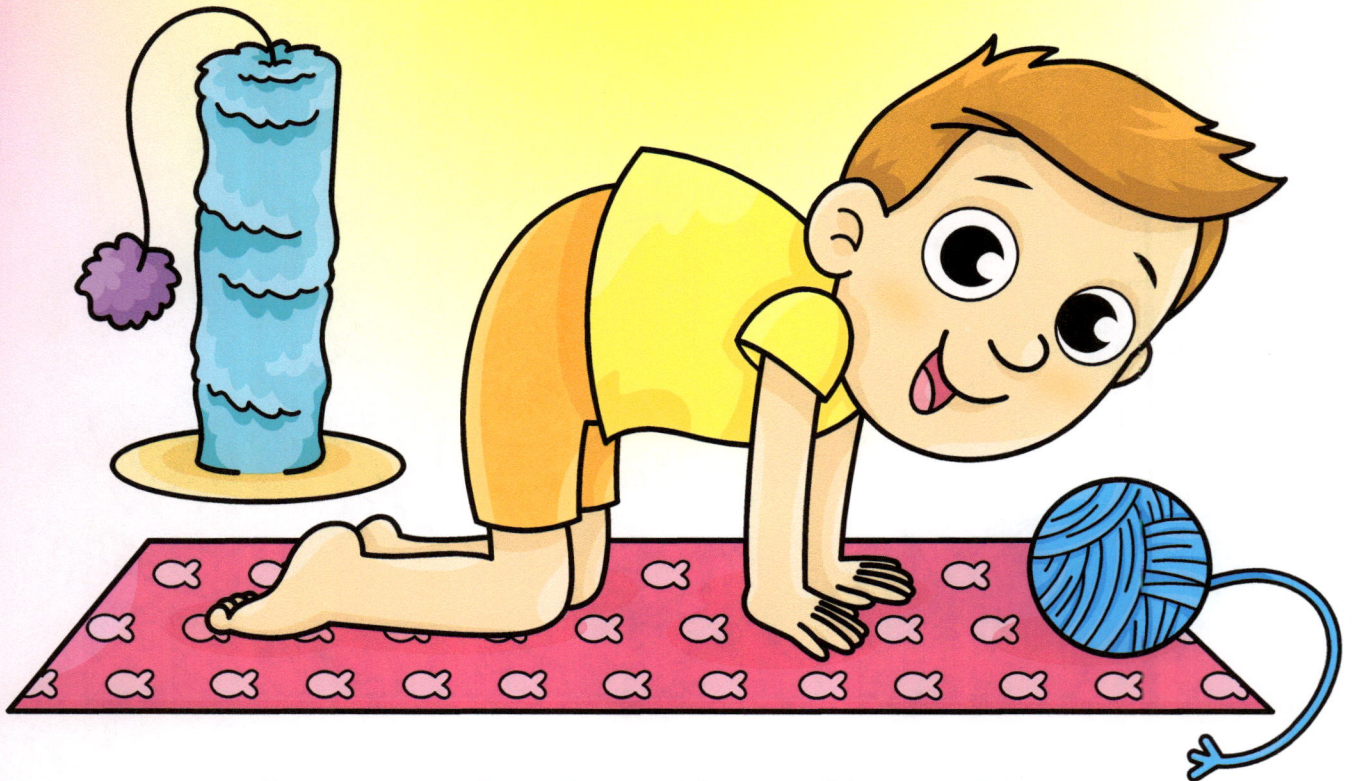

Go to your hands and knees like a table.
Then round your back and tuck your chin into your chest.

Can you "Meow" like a Cat?

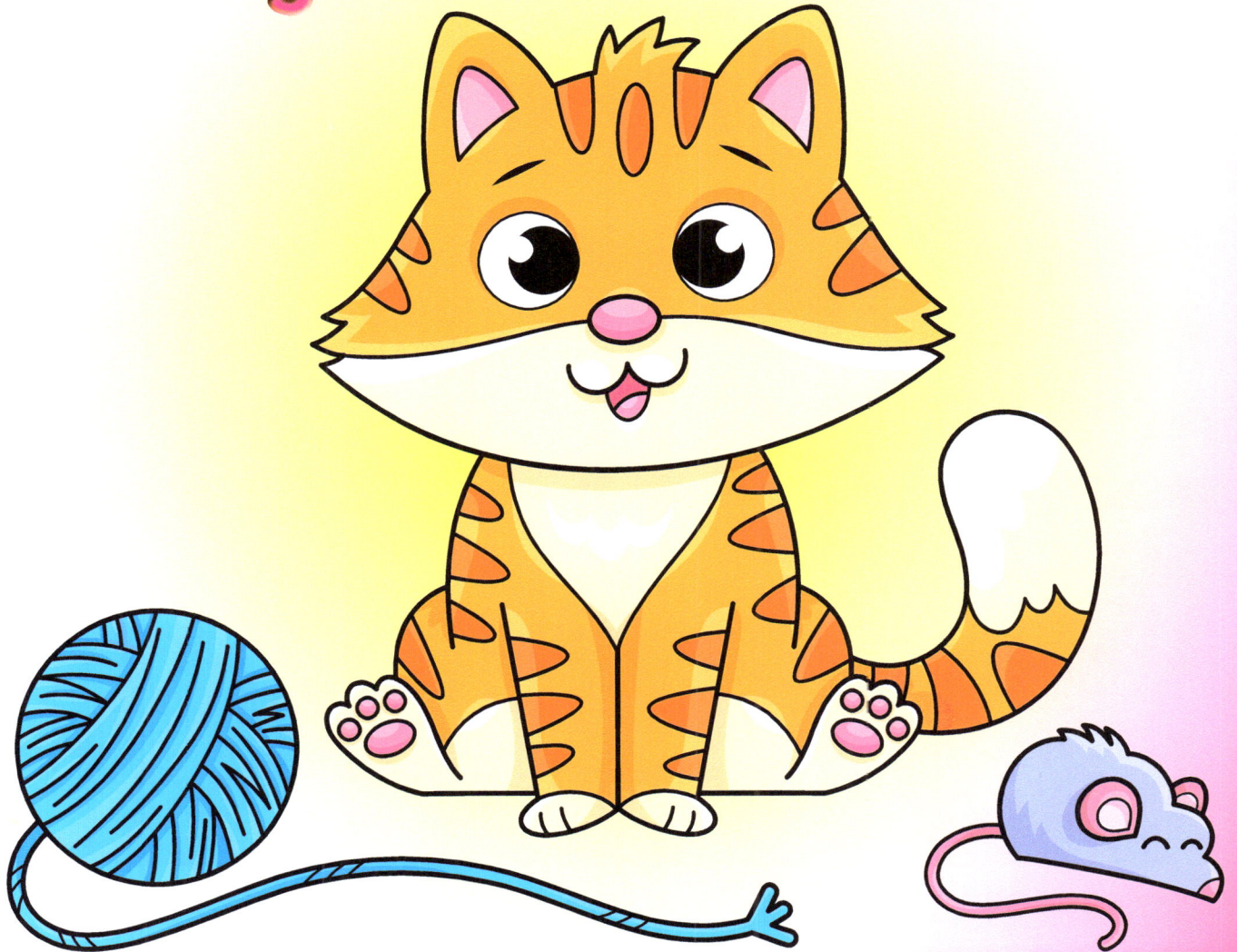

Their roaring is like a lion, like young lions they roar...
Isaiah 5:29 ESV

Cow

SHAPE

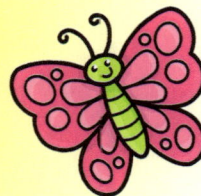

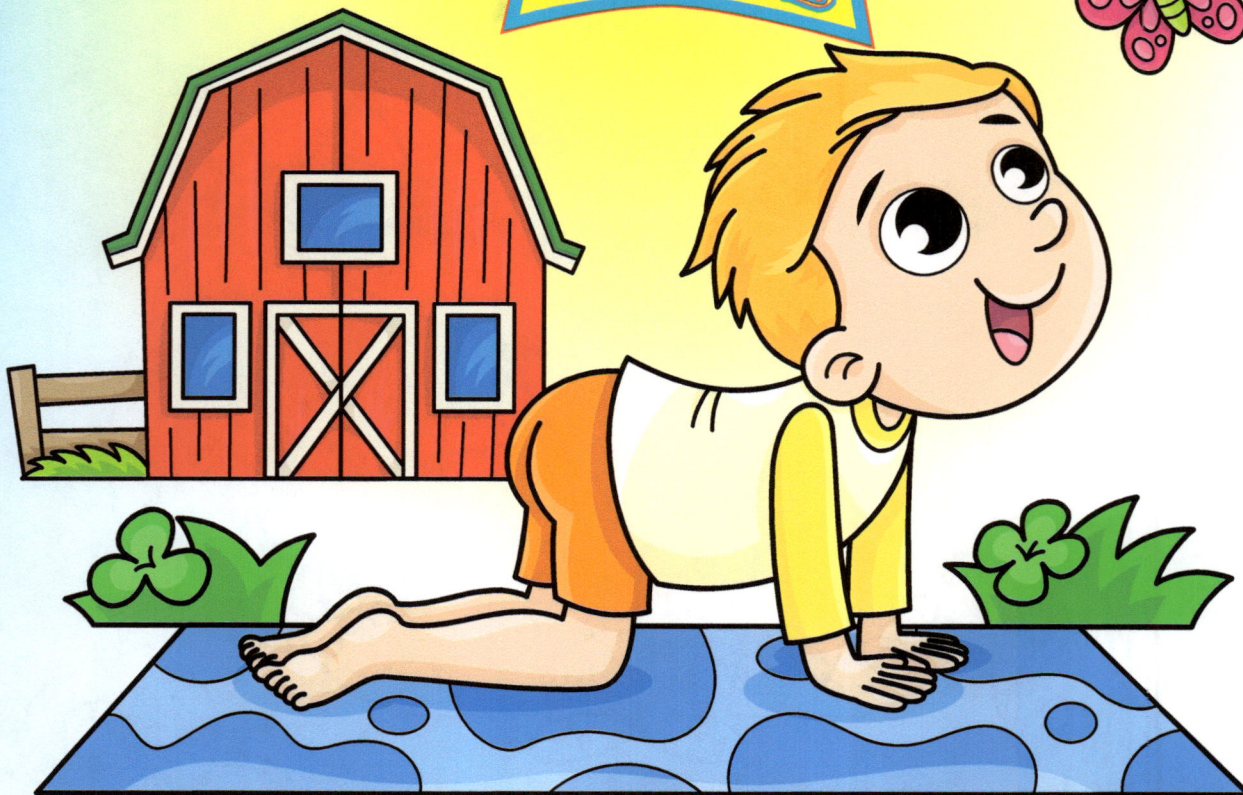

Come to a table on all fours
(hands and knees).
Then arch your back and look up.

Can you "Moo" like a Cow?

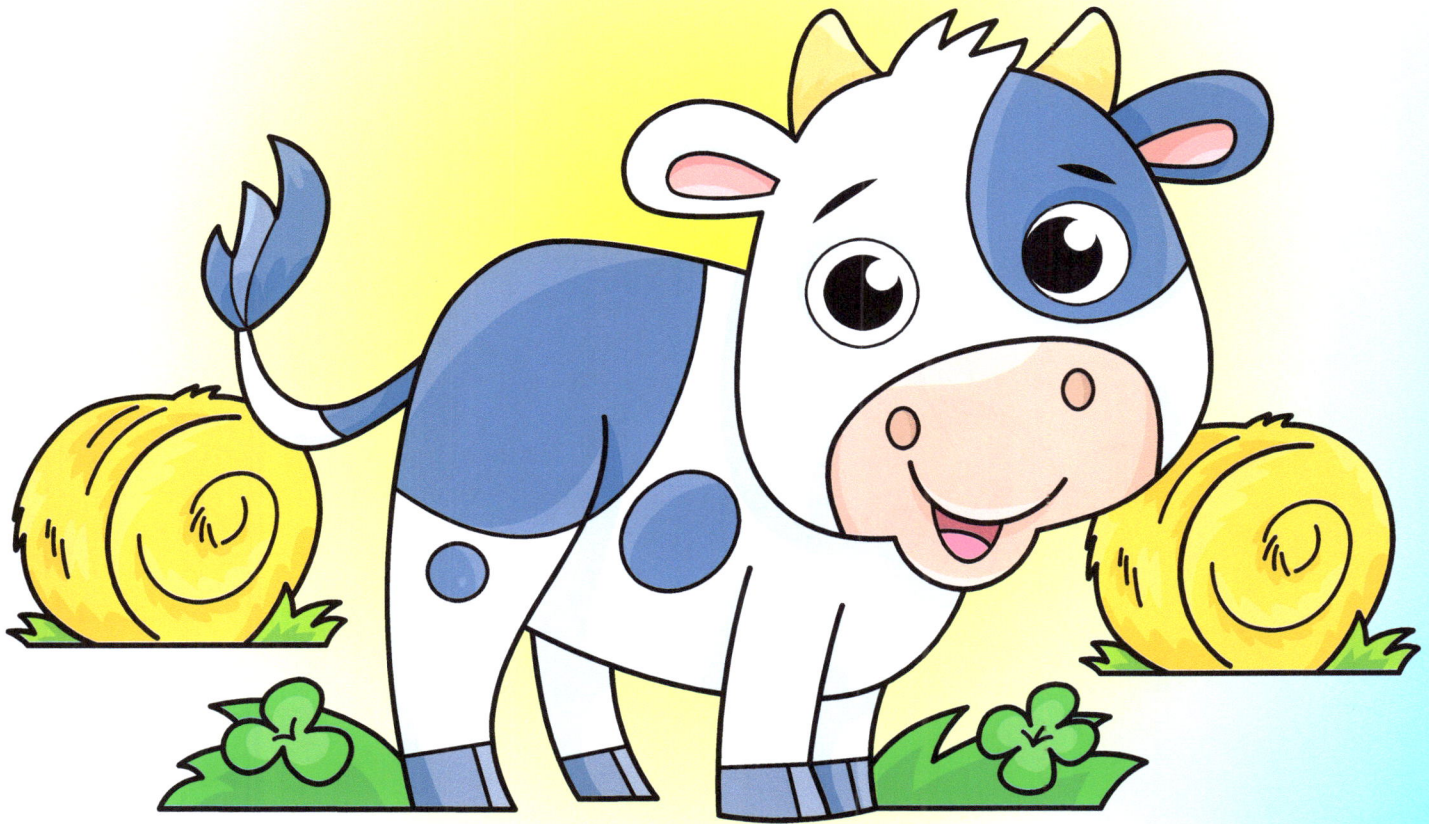

The cow and the bear shall graze;
their young shall lie down together.

Isaiah 11:6-9 ESV

Downward Dog

SHAPE

FIDO

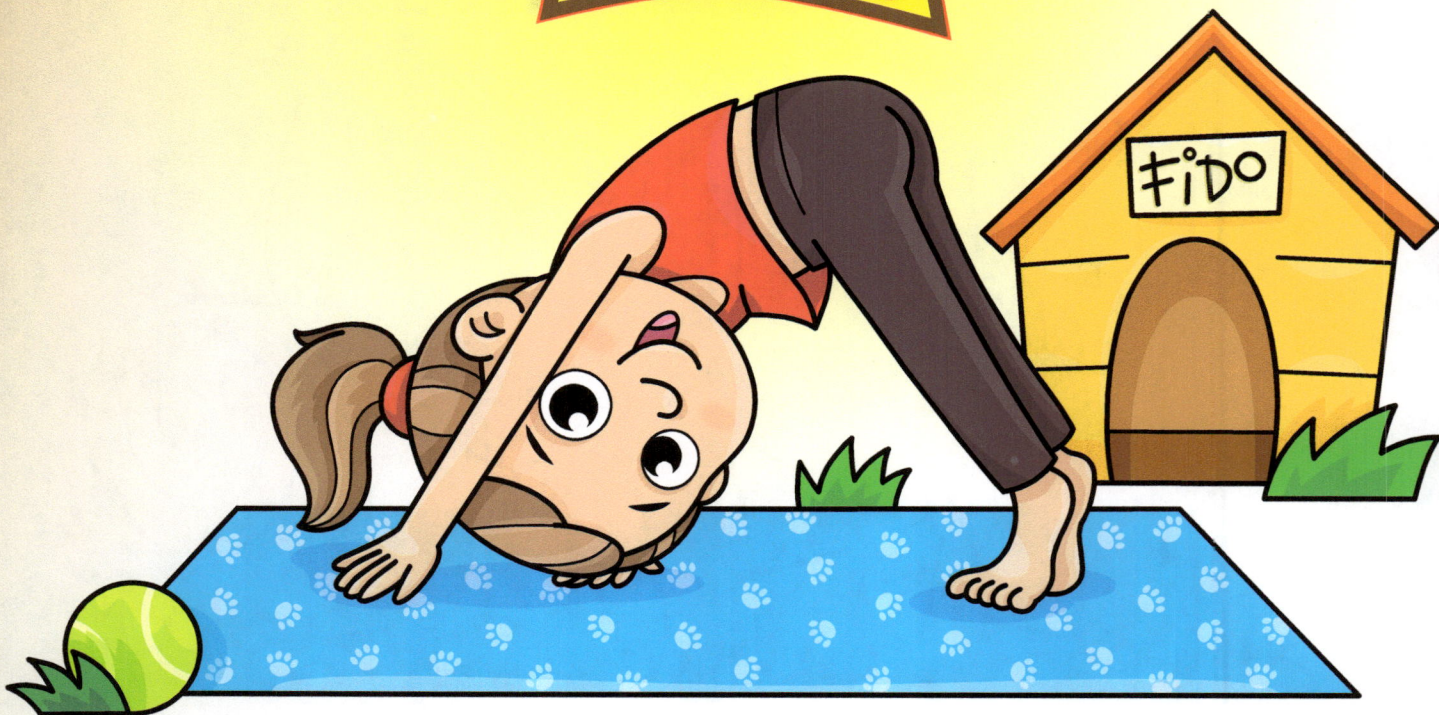

Put your palms flat on the floor and step your legs straight back.
Then relax your neck and head down, looking at the floor.
Your body looks like an upside down "V".

Can you "Bark" like a Dog?

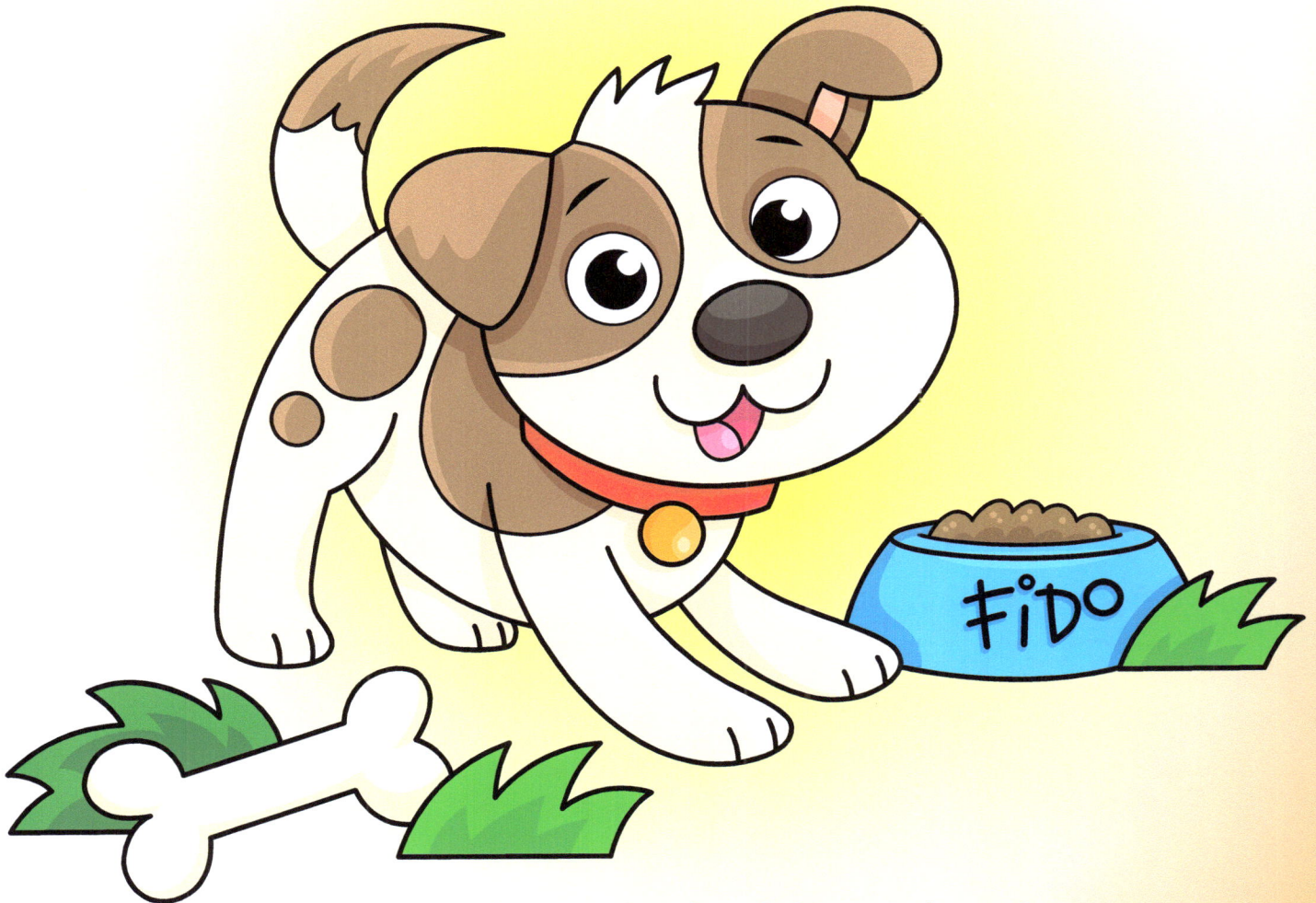

It is not right to take the children's bread
and throw it to the dogs.
Matthew 15:26 ESV

Dolphin

SHAPE

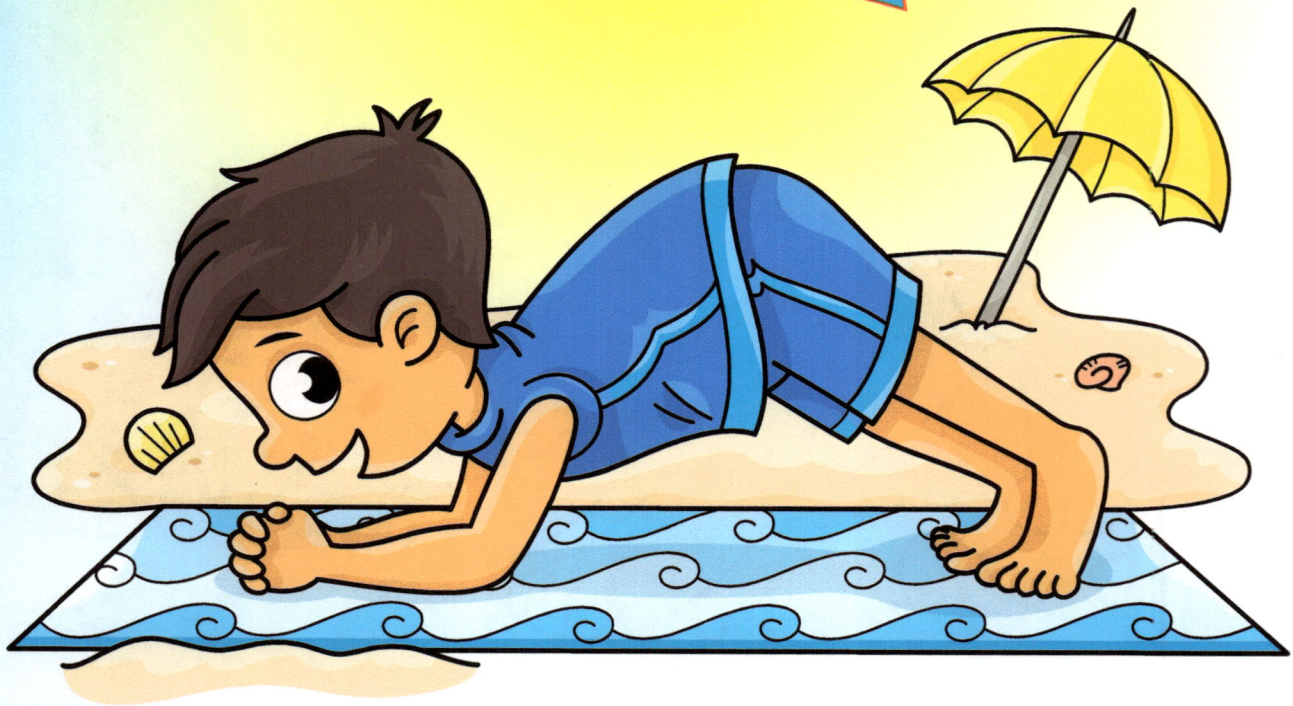

Bend your elbows and rest your forearms on the floor.
Then lift up your tailbone to the sky, and straighten them. Always look down.

Can you "Whistle" like a Dolphin?

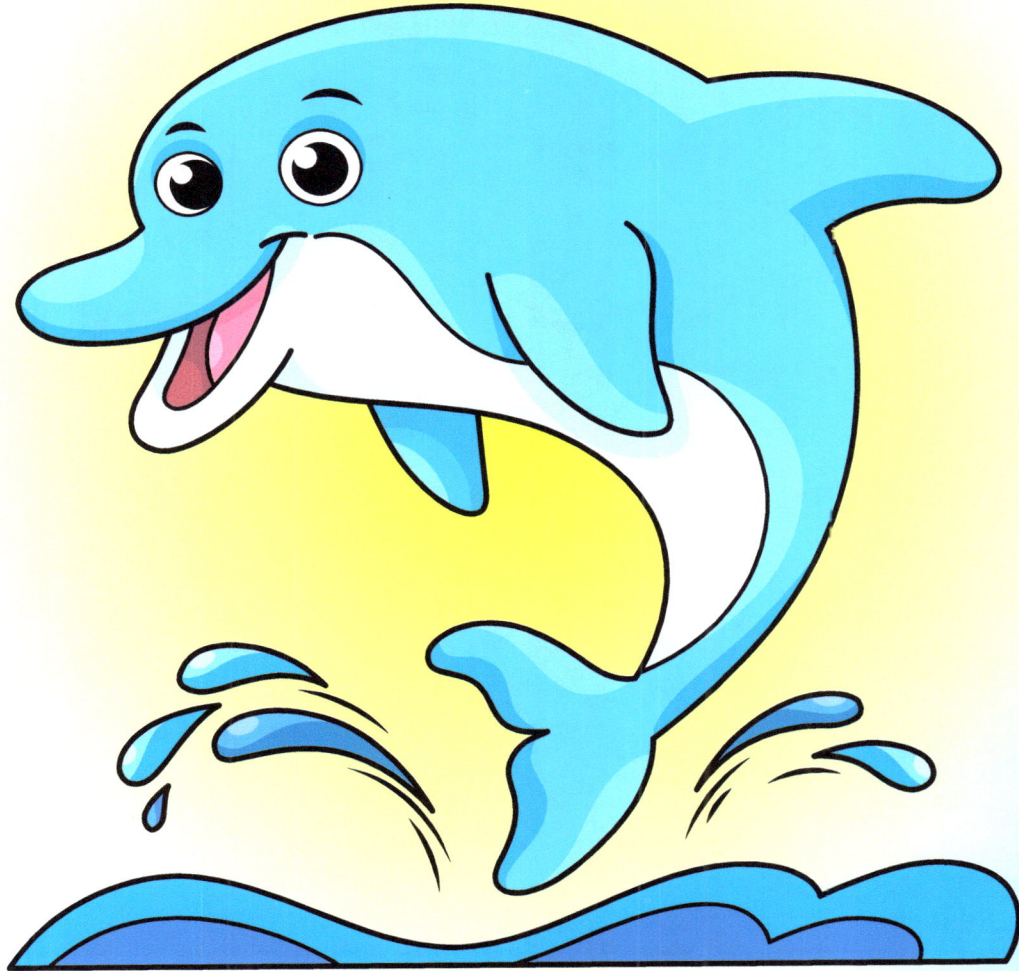

...and the fish in the sea,
all that swim the paths of the seas.
Psalm 8:8 NIV

Cobra

SHAPE

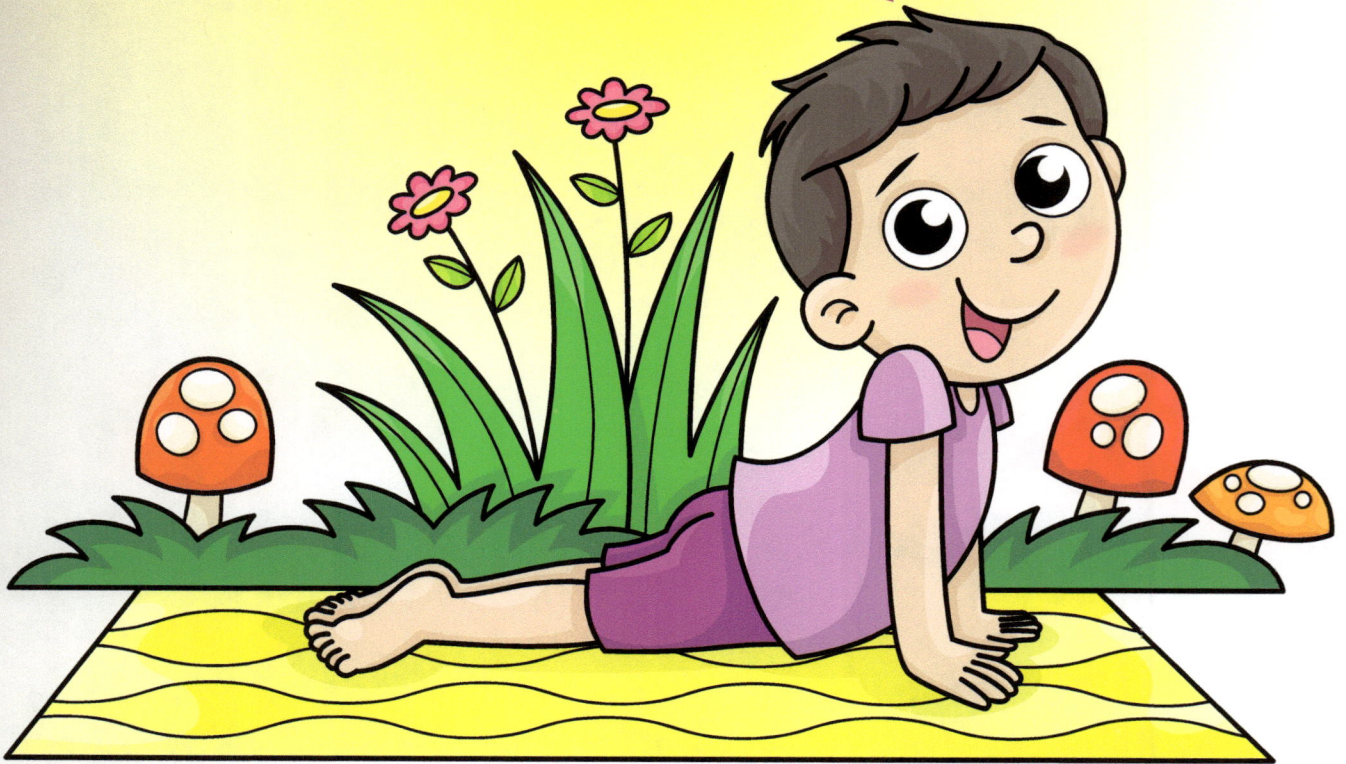

Lie on your stomach. Place your arms by your waist.
Then press into your hands by your ribs and lift your chest.

Can you "Hiss" like a Snake?

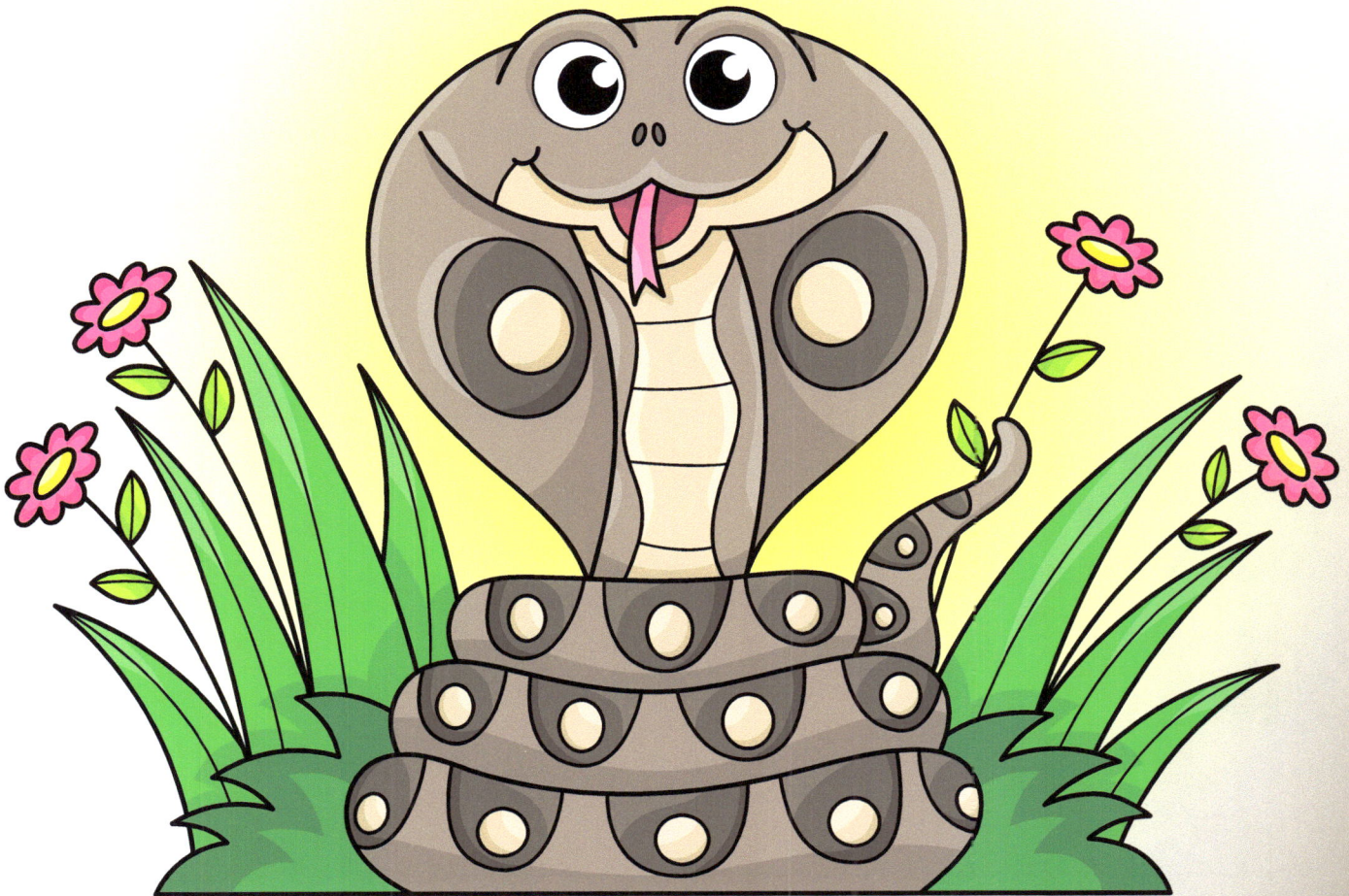

Just as Moses lifted up the snake in the
wilderness, so the Son of Man must be lifted up
John 3:14-15 NIV

Locust

SHAPE

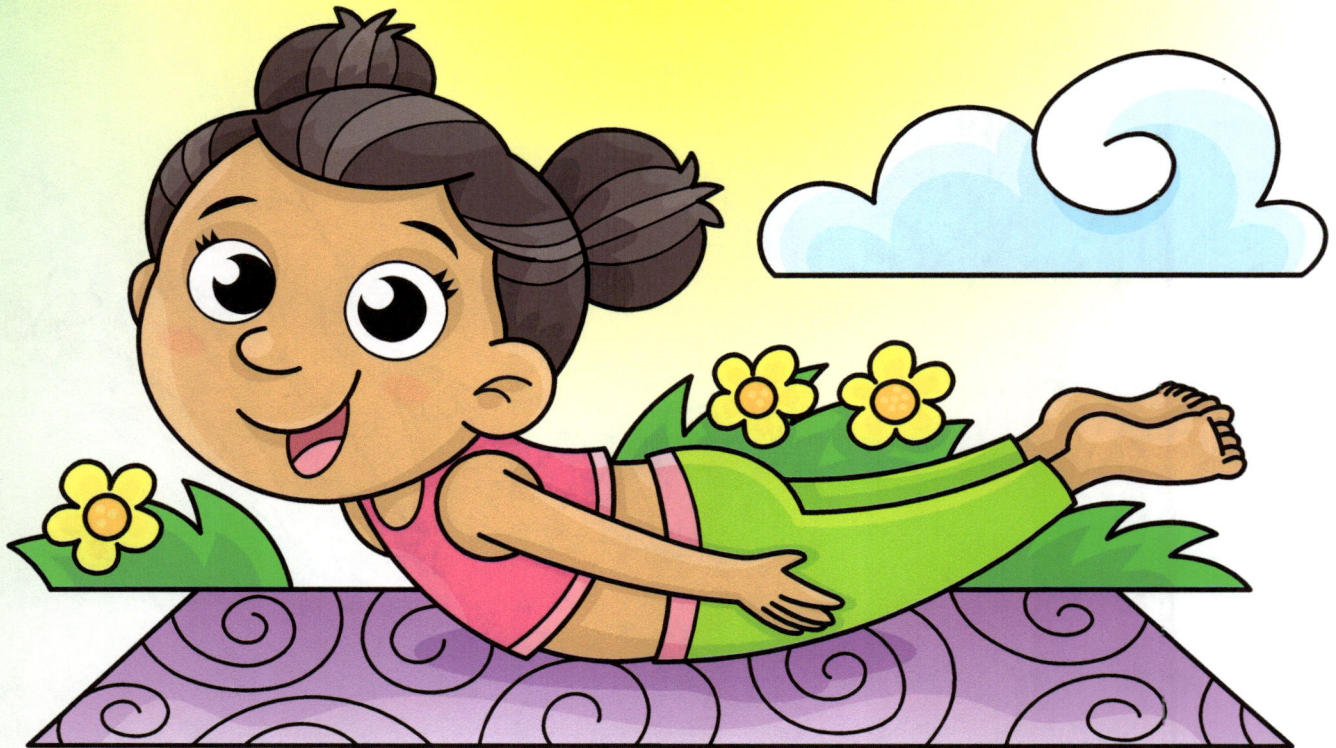

Lie on your stomach. Lift up your shoulders and chest.
Put your hands by your sides. Then lift both your legs up too.

Can you "Buzz" like a Locust?

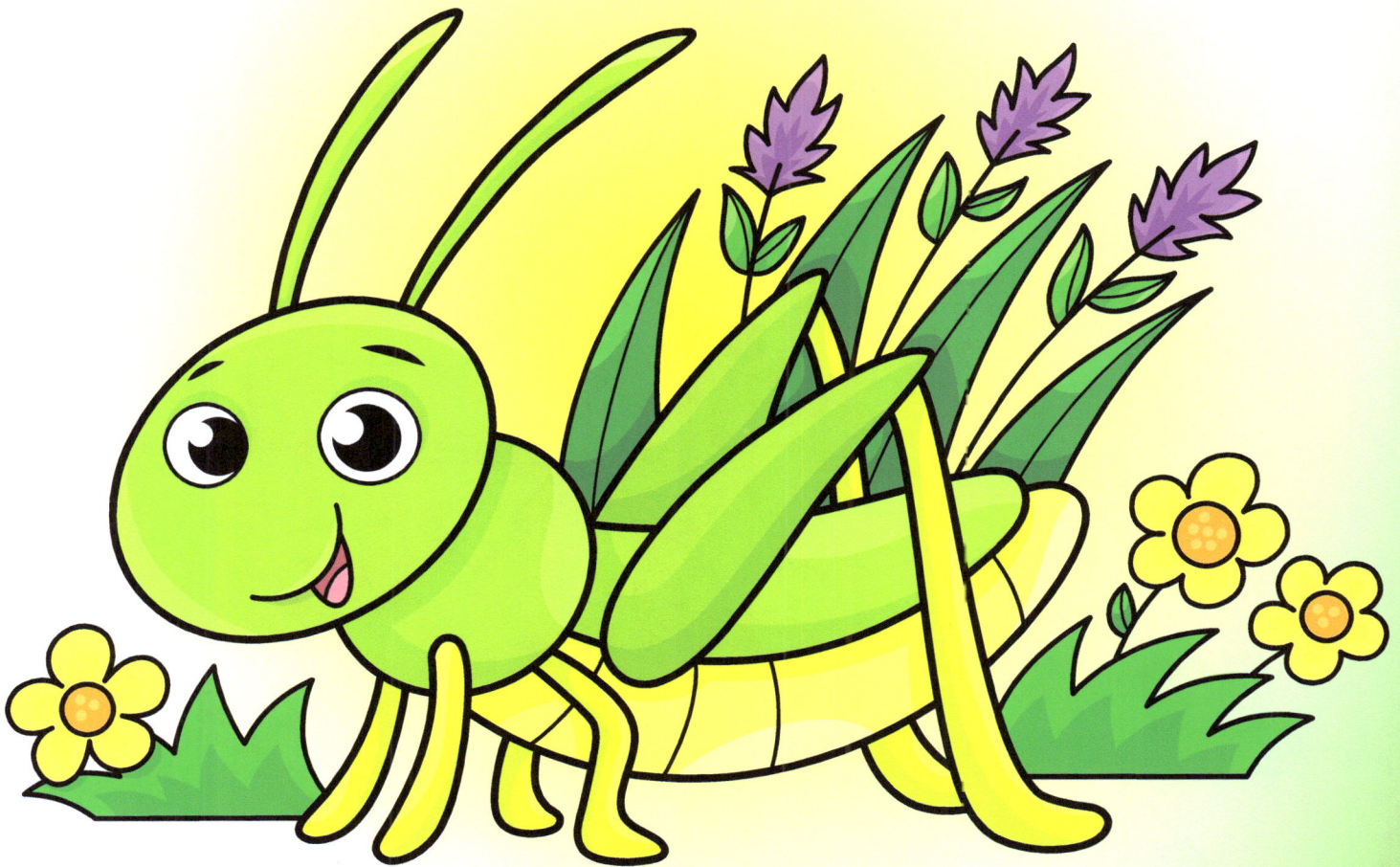

He spoke, and the locusts came,
young locusts without number
Psalm 105:34 ESV

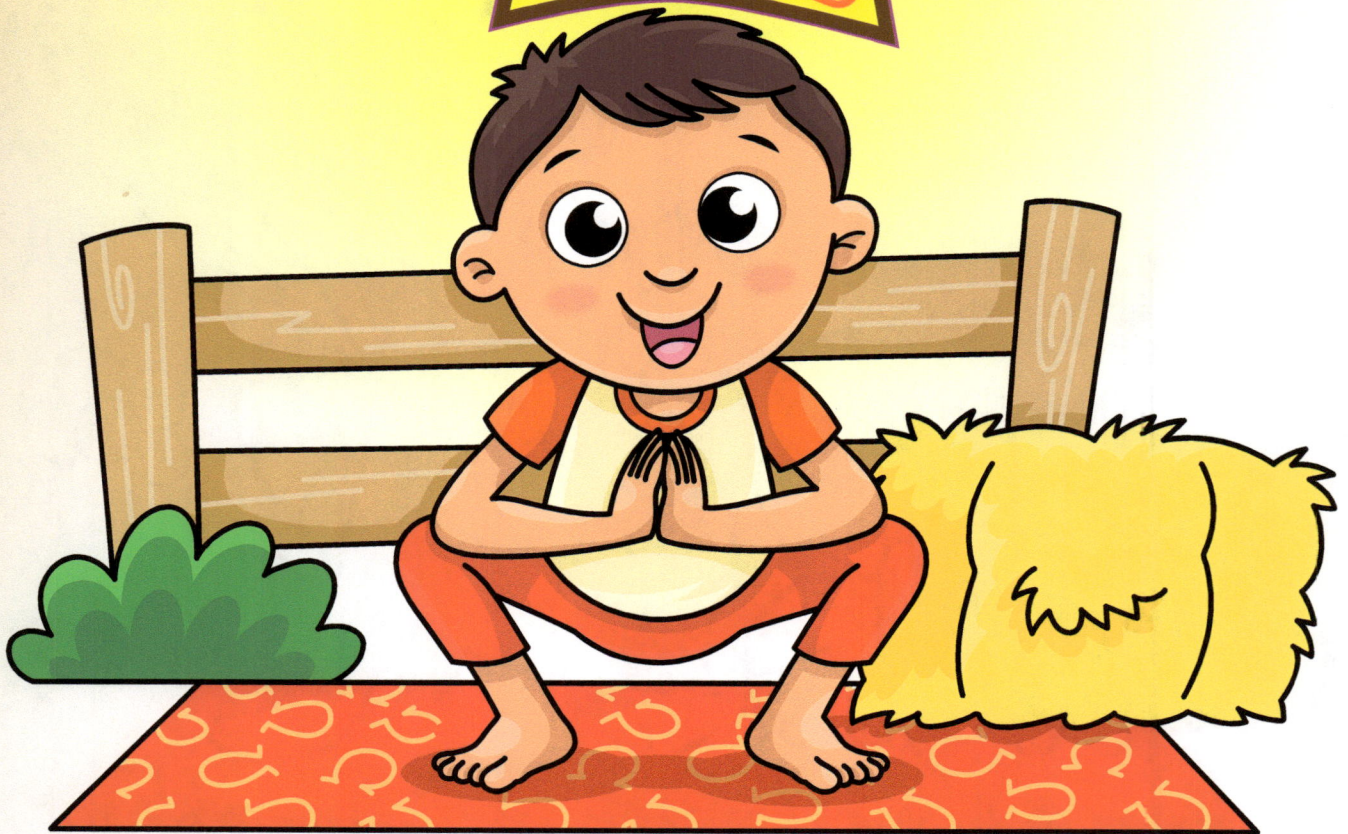

Horse
SHAPE

Put your legs apart with your feet facing outwards.
Bend your knees and fold your hands together.

Can you "Nay" like a Horse?

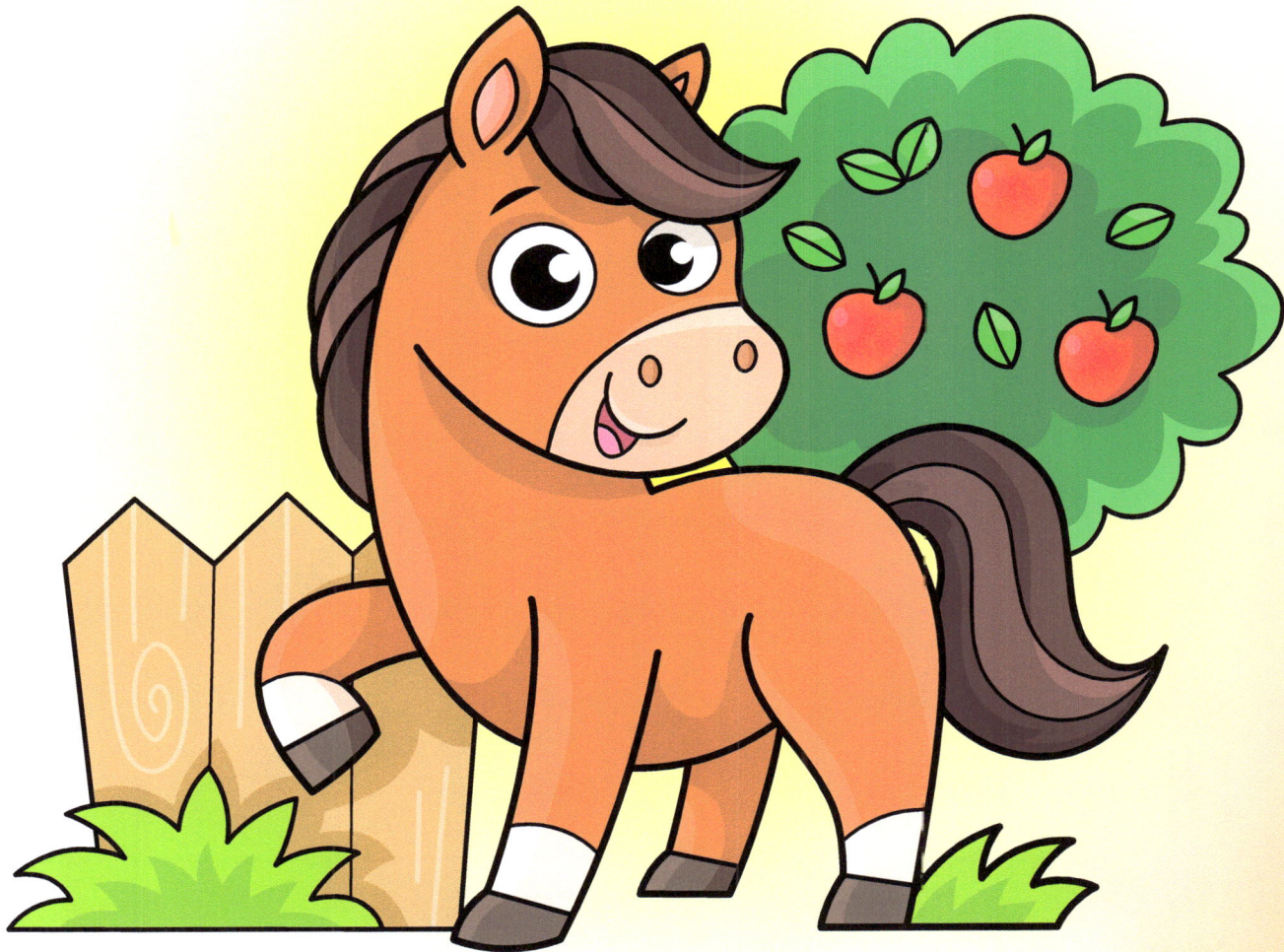

Solomon had four thousand stalls for chariot horses,
and twelve thousand horses.

1 Kings 4:26 NIV

Fish

SHAPE

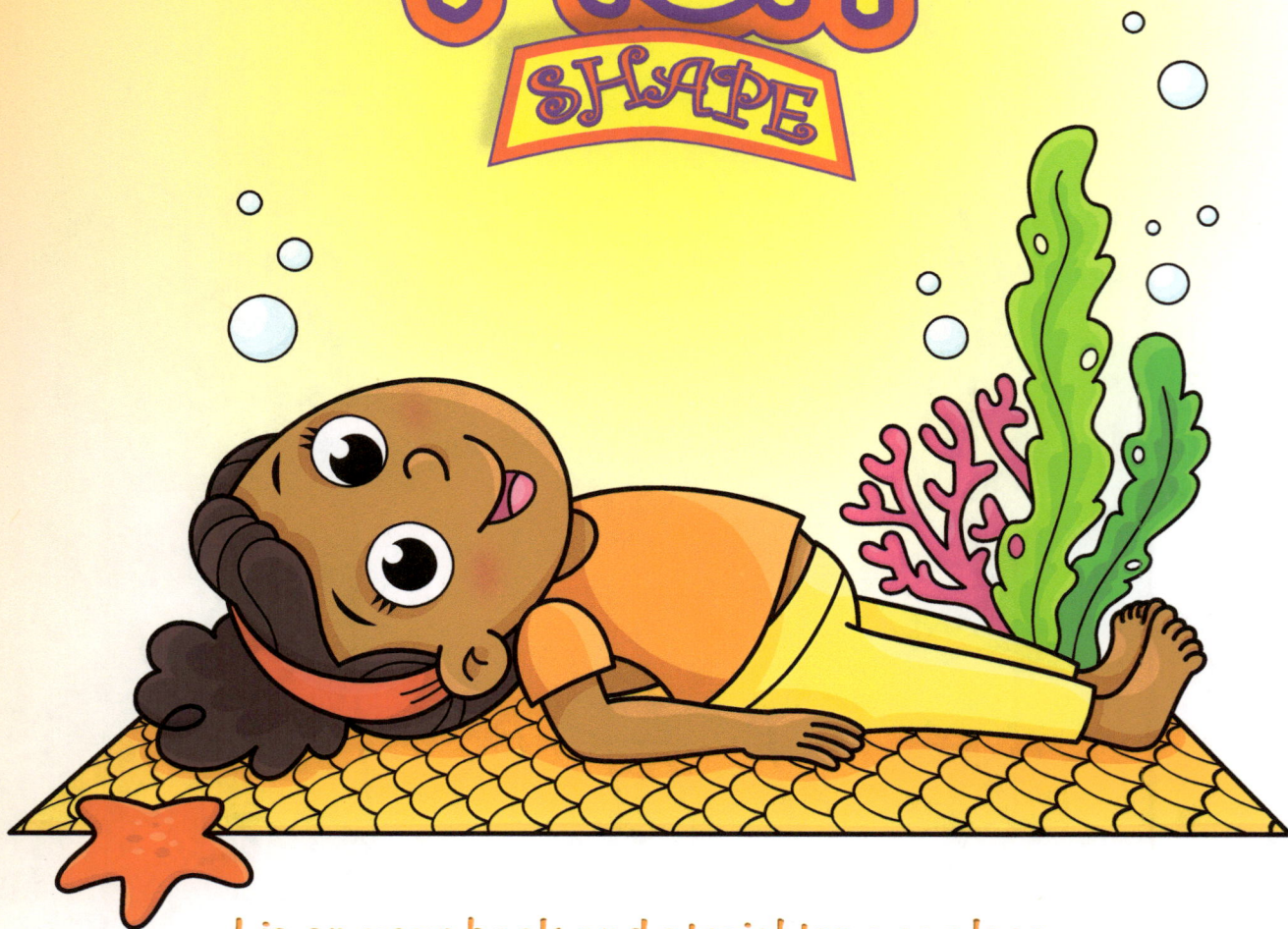

Lie on your back and straighten your legs.
Put your hands, palms facing down, under your bottom.
Then point your toes and come to the crown of your head.

Can you "Bubble" like a Fish?

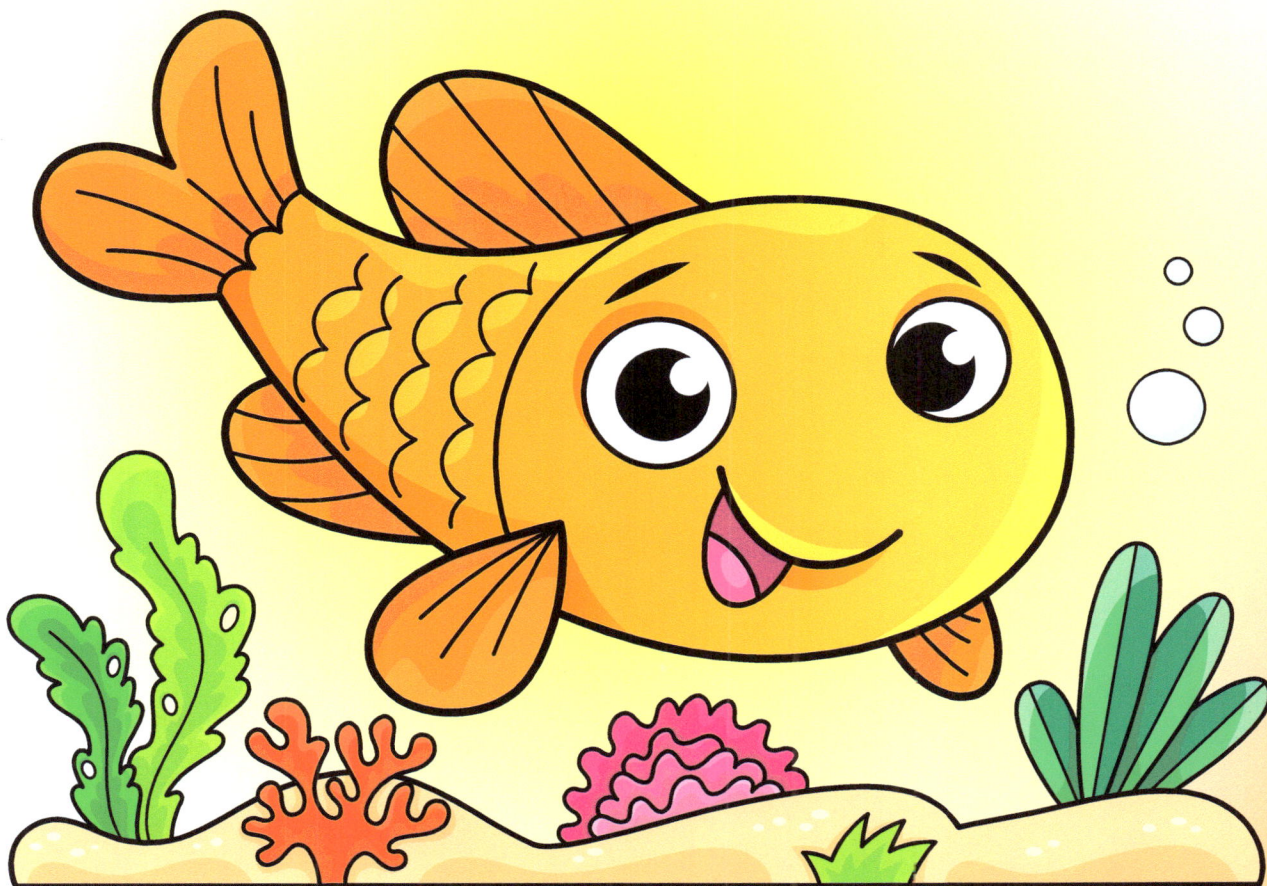

There will be a great many fish,
because this water will flow there and turn the salt water fresh.
Ezekiel 47:9 ISV

Godya™

This book title is intended
to be a series outlining
various yoga exercises
depicting all of
God's created works

About the Author

Linda Sakevich
is a physical education teacher
at a christian school.
She wants to introduce yoga to
children by combining her love
of teaching and yoga together,
through various bible verses.

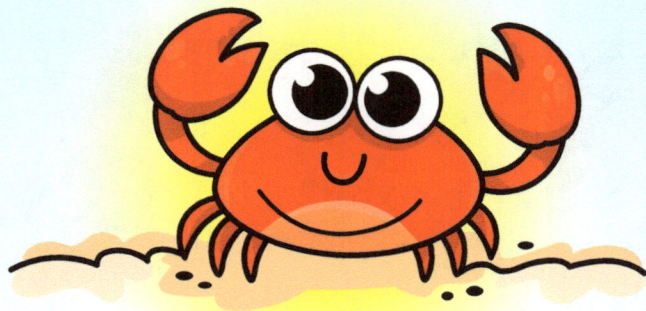

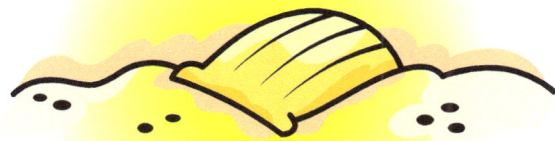

Godya™
God's Yoga for Kids

Animal Shapes

www.ingramcontent.com/pod-product-compliance
Lightning Source LLC
Chambersburg PA
CBHW061154030426
42336CB00002B/40